Mirror Madness
A Guide To Better Body Image
Mirror Madness A Guide To Better Body Image

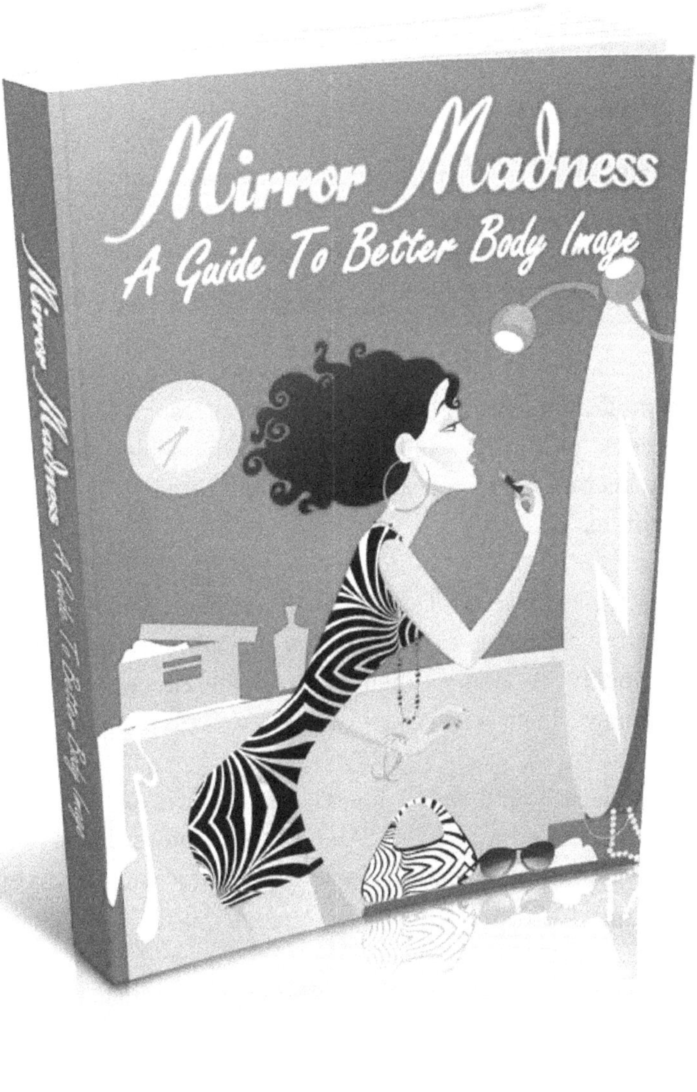

Terms and Conditions

Table Of Contents

Foreword

Body image is the representation we produce of what we think we look like; it might or may not bear a close relation to how other people really see us.

That is, they are subject to all sorts of distortion from inner elements like our emotions, moods, early experiences, mental attitudes of our parents, and much more.

All the same, it powerfully influences behavior. Engrossment with and distortions of body image are far-flung among American women , however they're driving forces in eating disorders, feeding severe panic than may be alleviated only by dieting. Get all the info you need here.

Mirror Madness
A Guide To Better Body Image

Chapter 1:

Body Image Basics

Synopsis

Tired of fretting about the way you look? Read this.

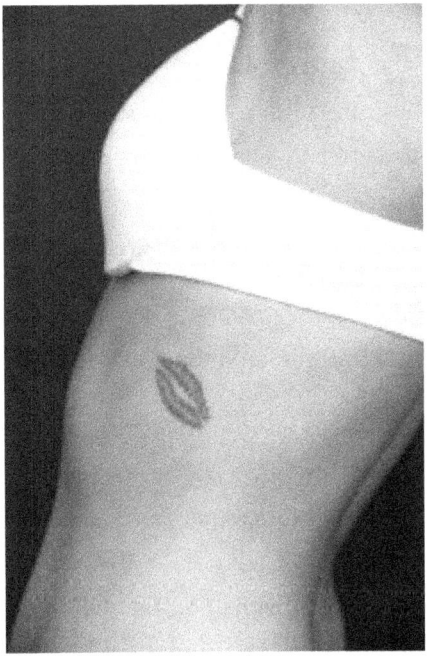

The Basics

Utilizing methods from cosmetic surgery to miracle diets to liposuction, women in increasing numbers are endeavoring-with a degree of panic and, more frequently than not, to their own harm-to match the elemental template of beauty.

Has the state of affairs declined in the past few decades? The reply is undeniably yes. Men, too, no longer appear immune.

In 1987 a survey about appearance and weight revealed that only 12 % of those polled indicated little concern about their look and said they didn't do much to better it. The results of this survey are similar to those of a lot of studies where the participants are chosen at random: individuals feel intense pressure to look great.

Weight has become so important to body image; it's the focus of dissatisfaction in both studies and the area demonstrating the biggest increase.

Body engrossment has become a social mania. We've become a land of appearance junkies and fitness partisans, pioneers driven to think, talk, strategize, and fret about our bodies with the same fanatic devotion we gave to putting a man on the moon. Overseas, we strive for global peace. At home, we have announced war on our bodies.

Of all the industrial accomplishments of the 20th century that influence how we view our bodies, none has had a heavier effect than the rise of the mass media. With movies, magazines, and TV, we see beautiful individuals as frequently as we see our own family members; the net effect is to make great beauty seem real and gettable.

A lot of women avoid the mirror totally; those who do look might scrutinize, yet all the same fail to see themselves objectively. Most of us see only afflictive flaws in keen detail. Other people still see the fat and flaws that used to be there in the adolescent years, even if they're no longer there.

A woman today views her reflection in a mirror and finds it wanting-- and then is devoured by a pursuit to make herself fit the reflection the mass media has conditioned her to anticipate is conceivable. She works harder and harder to gain what is most likely inconceivable. Brushing aside the hours movie stars spend on makeup and hair, forgetting how simply and well the camera may lie, she aspires to a man-made composite of what she thinks her reflection ought to be.

We might be heavy and think that life isn't worth living as we don't match our culture's physical ideal. Our self-image has become way too plastic, too tactile.

It counts too much on passing moods, on what we feel is expected of us and how we feel we are lacking. It isn't subject enough to an unchanging inner sense of ourself. We grow bigger or smaller, in our mind's eye, in reaction to the image of woman modern order has promoted us to idealize.

We're stuck in a world of obsessive self-criticism, where what we see isn't at all what we truly are. The mirror is woman's modern curse.

A few call such obsession with appearance conceit-however that misses the point. We're responding to the deep psychological meaning of the body. Appearance does indeed impact our sense of self and how individuals react to us; it always has, always will. What's different nowadays is that the body and how it looks has gotten to be a substantial part of our self-worth.

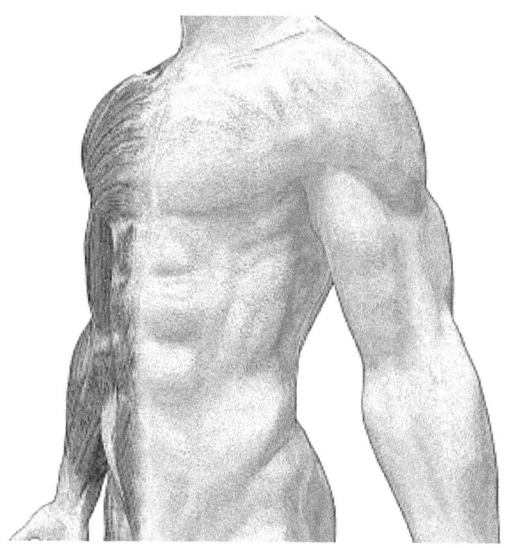

Chapter 2:

Learn To Love Yourself

Synopsis

Do you love yourself? This is a query that might appear simple, yet a lot of individuals have a hard time answering it. There's nothing wrong in loving yourself. Loving yourself is essential for your well being. Loving yourself is essential to lead a successful and happy life filled with confidence. After all, how may you become happy if you don't love yourself? As happiness comes from inside, you have to love yourself in the process.

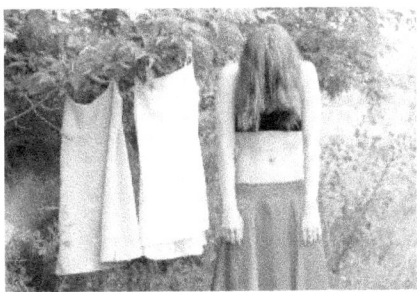

Self Love

Take care with your self talk. Learn to talk to yourself in a favorable and loving way. A lot of individuals talk negatively to themselves and keep saying things like "I'm not good" "I won't accomplish my goals." "I'm depressed" among extra statements.

If you talk positively to yourself, you're programming your subconscious with positive images. Whatever you program your subconscious with is what you draw in to your life. Begin speaking kindly to yourself and you'll be on the path to self love.

Forgive yourself. I'm sure you've made some errors that you're not proud of. Understand that we all make errors. There's no individual that hasn't made errors in life.

There are a few individuals who made errors and keep feeling guilty. They believe they can't and should not be forgiven. What you have to remember is that there's nothing that you've done that you shouldn't be forgiven for.

Forgiving yourself could take a little time, however if you learn to alter your thoughts and view the errors you've done as experiences that you learn from, forgiving yourself will be much simpler for you.

Always love yourself. A lot of individuals begin to lose confidence in themselves if they come across somebody who doesn't like them. Let me ask you a question, do you like and get along with everybody that you come across in life?

Life is filled with individuals who have assorted views and beliefs about different situations, cultures, politics and faith. It's that difference that makes life beautiful and satiated with different opportunities.

You have to like yourself at all times. You're a precious present to the world. Learn to love yourself categorically. Differentiate between who you are and your behaviors. Love yourself for the simple fact that you live.

Spoil yourself. Learn to spoil yourself with something you love. Spoiling and treating yourself helps reduce your tension and worry. When you're free of tension and worry, your brain is quiet and you're able to love yourself more freely.

Quit seeking approval. If you're like most individuals, the chances are you sought-after approval at one time in life. It's great to want individual's approval, but when approval gets to be a need rather than a want, this is when it gets dangerous and might affect your self love.

Not seeking approval is great for you as it teaches you to be confident in yourself and in your values. There are a lot of individuals who put a lot of importance on what others say. While listening to what others say is significant, their view shouldn't be more significant than your view. Remember, you're a unique individual that ought to always be loved. You're a true present to the world and don't ever forget that.

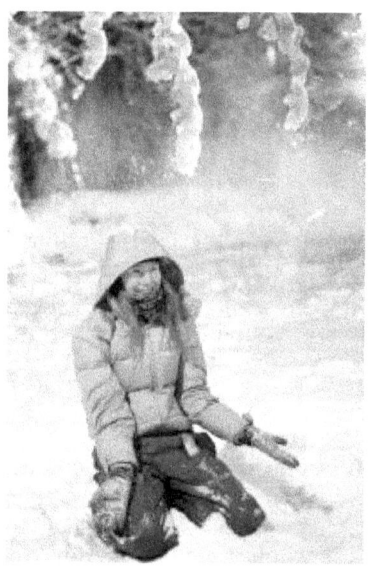

Chapter 3:

Get Involved In A Sport You Love

Synopsis

We live in a cultivation which celebrates slenderness and condemns fatness. For young women, the fear of-becoming fat formulates during adolescence and goes on into adulthood, even among slender, active females.

These fears may produce patterns of over-exercise or under-eating which might have devastating health outcomes. Poor intakes of food and calcium may lead to osteoporosis (bone-thinning), and a low calorie consumption may contribute to amenorrhoea (lack of normal menses), which, by lowering the output of the bone-building sex hormone oestrogen, may increase the severity of osteoporosis.

Extreme engrossment with thinness may likewise lead to anorexia nervosa and/or bulimia, two disorders which may produce an array of ruinous physical issues.

Using Articles

What's the most beneficial way for young women to better their perceptions of their bodies and hopefully lower their risk of formulating anemia, anorexia, bulimia and osteoporosis?

According to researchers, participation in sports is among the best body-image enhancers. Researchers studied 152 young women of age 11-17 who were attending summer programs, both in the U.S. and Mexico. The young women filled in questionnaires designed to get info about perceived weight, worries about weight, dieting behavior, body image, and components shaping body image.

Researchers likewise measured each young lady's BMI (Body Mass Index). The young women in the study reflected their culture's idolization of slenderness, tending to overestimate their weight if they were of a normal weight and being pleased if they were skinny. For instance, women who saw themselves as too fat really had a healthy weight/height ratio. Teenagers who had high body image had a BMI below-normal.

Sports involvement was linked with bettered body image. Young women who played on greater numbers of sports teams had greater body images, likened to women who played on few or no squads.

Aside from sports involvement, the material but not the frequency of parental remarks was likewise vital in determining body image. Body image marks of young women who got negative comments from parents were much tougher than the self-ratings of women who got favorable comments.

Overall, women with high body image tended not to look outside themselves to specify their body images; inside they were able to get feelings of self worth which extended to their physical looks.

Why did sports involvement assist body image? It's thought that sports-team involvement may be a source of self-pride through approval from peers, parents, and acquaintances. The young women in the study likewise reported that team participation helped make them feel that their bodies were 'able' and 'competent'.

These favorable feelings seemed to produce a moderately high level of gratification with their bodies.

Chapter 4:

Stop Comparing Yourself To Others

Synopsis

Comparing is an innate tendency we all have. It may be utterly neutral, as if you simply evaluate similarities and differences. Such comparing is necessary for astute reasoning.

It's likewise productive if you're prompted to emulate someone's impressive traits. But, it becomes dysfunctional when it conjures up the green-eyed monster and jealousy, if you label yourself as better as or less than other people.

Consider it: Without comparisons, jealousy and the green-eyed monster could not exist. Interestingly, it's more common to feel deficient to those with "more" than to feel thankful compared to those with "less."

Be Happy With You

We're a fellowship of comparison addicts. It begins from day one. Children are compared to one another. Who's smarter, more precious? Then comes elementary school. Not so different from the breakdown of our comparisons in later life, interpersonally and politically.

Comparing yourself to other people may prevent a bond of common companionship and is a disservice to discovering true worth. Either you'll wind up with the short end of the stick or, if you put yourself above anybody, you're nowhere. (No one is above anybody else.) Self-pride must come from merely being you.

Pick out an individual you feel jealousy or the green-eyed monster towards. Maybe a colleague your supervisor prefers. Or a cocky, well-off relation. Make this individual your test case prior to you going on to transform these emotions with other people.

Act differently. Rehearse dealing with jealousy and the green-eyed monster by heedfully utilizing humility and preventing comparisons, even if the individual irritates you. For example, instead of mechanically bristling or shrinking in your seat when your supervisor praises this colleague, 2nd her great ideas, a collegial reaction.

Attempt not to feed into feeling "less than." Rather, as an endowed equal, add your own great ideas, not letting their resonance or your shaky self-pride discourage you. Though you've the right to be distressed about your supervisor's favoritism, a modest but positive approach will begin to better things. In this instance and the situation with your prosperous relation, practice the precept "I shall not compare." Switch your mentality to center on what you do have, what makes you satisfied. Let that be the tone of your fundamental interaction.

Give to other people what you most want for yourself. If you need your work to be treasured, treasure other people' work. If you need love, give love. If you need a successful profession, help another's profession to flourish. What gets around comes around.

Learn from a competitors favorable points. Get your brain off of what you perceive you lack and toward self-reformation. Transform the green-eyed monster to appreciation, and what you look up to will become part of your life.

Wish a competitor well. Even if it's difficult to accomplish this, try. It helps you to turn negativism around to something more favorable.

Enlisting these techniques helps you take your eyes off of others and back to yourself. The point is to apprize what you have instead of center on what you're lacking. A huge part of emotional freedom is developing self-compassion instead of beating yourself up.

Praise yourself. Gain self-pride from your efforts to deal with the green-eyed monster or positively. Demonstrating humbleness and putting off comparisons lets you build self-pride. It nurtures a loving versus defensive attitude in relationships.

Chapter 5:

Wear The Right Clothes

Synopsis

It's a huge deal that your clothes affect or influence other people. However what about selecting the correct clothes so that they best affect you?

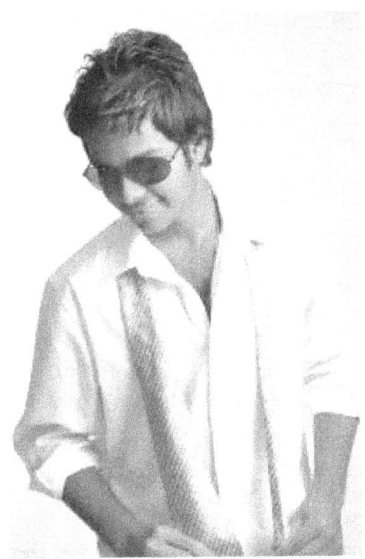

The Right Stuff

A lately published study by 2 educatees supplies insights into how to get the correct mentality by selecting the correct clothes. They produced the term "enclothed cognition" to distinguish a procedure that impacts your mentality based on the symbolic meaning and the tangible experience of wearing your clothes.

They did a series of experimentations to test their hypothesis, by utilizing a lab coat. In one trial, players wearing a lab coat were seen to have a sense of enhanced regard.

A 2nd trial had players wearing the same laboratory coat, which was identified as it being a physician's coat. In the 3rd trial, participants were told that the coat was a coat for a painter.

Those wearing the physicians coat demonstrated a higher level of maintained attention as likened to those thought to be donning a painter's coat.

So, one takeaway from this experimentation is that if your mends are wearing doctor's coats, they're more probable to be more thoughtful, and even more careful.

Most of us don't don lab coats, or any coat for that matter. How may this experimentation help you to get the correct mindset by selecting the correct clothes?

One common denominator for nearly everybody I know is denim. Let's look at an illustration that you'll easily relate to.

One of my customers, a successful enterpriser, told me just last week how he's in jeans 7 days a week now. He outwears jeans for business meetings, to church service, and everyplace in between.

However he requires a particular sort of denim jean to wear when he works on his auto or while doing yard work. He wouldn't wear those jeans to lounge around in the home.

So those jeans have to have a dissimilar look and feel so he may wear them in an unstrained way. Then, for business meetings and for church service, another level of jeans would be more suitable.

If you required clothes to wear for similar conditions in your own life, and if wearing jeans was to be central to your every day wardrobe, every different sort of denim would help you to be in the correct mentality.

If my customer is wearing the sort of jeans to work on the auto or in the yard, he may feel like he may get into his work and may get those jeans as filthy as necessary. He wouldn't wear them to loaf around in the home or to business meetings as they might be soiled from that work.

Even if the auto and yard denims were clean, he'd know that those are purely for doing harder work. That's why it's crucial to his mentality to have another selection of denim for those meetings and for church service. More than being disrespectful to other people to look like he just crept out from under his auto, wearing those grimy jeans would very likely impact his thinking and behavior at a business meeting or at church service.

Here's my hint: When viewing the clothes in your closet, stop and think about how picking out the correct clothes will help you acquire the correct mentality first, then decide what you're going to wear, and how come you're going to wear it.

Your clothes don't just wire messages to other people. You select one item over another because of your mission for that day. Making favorable wardrobe selections prove that selecting the correct clothes influences your energy state and your thinking.

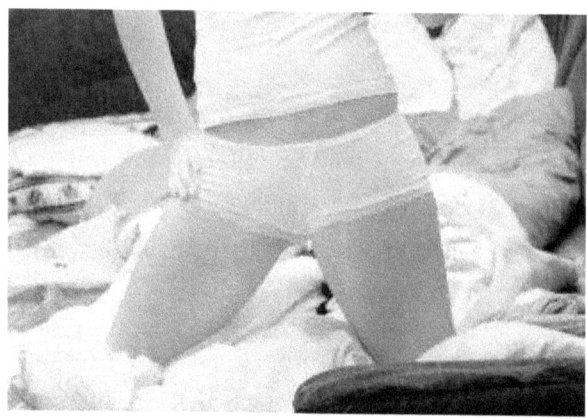

Chapter 6:

The Dangers Of Poor Body Image

Synopsis

The accompanying are the risks of a bad body image:

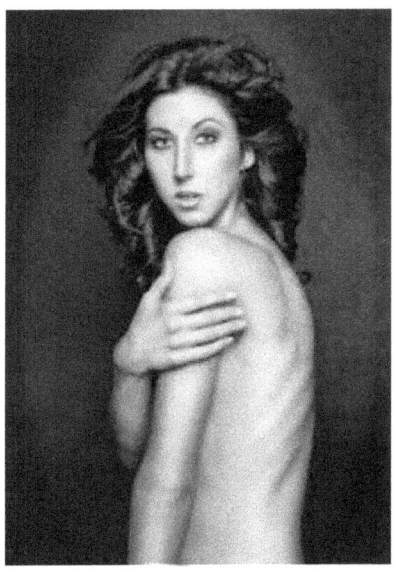

The Risks

•Potential for ill health (like eating disorders, or compulsive working out).
•Diminished self-pride.
•Lessening in drive to succeed.
•Inability to treasure one's self.
•Diminished confidence.

Most of the risks of a bad body image reside under the subject of merely not being able to see yourself for what you truly are. If when you look in the mirror you simply see what is amiss with you, that transfers into extra areas of your life.

It's hard to be satisfied, find a great job, have a fit relationship, or be successful in your attempts, regardless what they are, if you can't have a true grasp on yourself. You have to be able to have a cognizance of your value and your worth, and a bad body image ruins that.

It ruins self-assurance. It ruins motivation. And frequently, it not only cramps these matters but it may likewise create serious hurdles to defeat also.

For instance, it may lead to eating disorders which cause grave risk to your health, psychological issues, and frequently take years to defeat, and some never get over all of the effects. The risks of a bad body image are true, and shouldn't be taken lightly.

So, what may you do to help your girls have a favorable body image?

Begin with yourself. If you don't practice what you preach it will have little effect. Never talk badly about your own body in front of your girls. If you're shopping, and you call back you look bad, say, "This is the incorrect cut for me." Don't state, "Ugg, I look atrocious in this."

Help them formulate talents. Individuals who have developed their talents and realize their own talents tend to have more self-assurance then others. If you are able to support the growth in your youngsters, encourage them to follow their dreams, and formulate their talents, they'll feel valued, and will likely have less conflict with their body.

Nurture feelings of self worth. Supply an accepting environment that values differences in views and thoughts. Help your youngsters feel their place in your life, and their value to you. Helping your daughter feel self worth in additional areas of life will help her to feel worthwhile even if her body isn't perfect.

Speak positively. Don't say bad things about your body or anybody else's. Don't compare individuals based upon physical stature. Don't compare yourself or anybody else to a celebrity or super model. They pay to have exceptional bodies, work out a lot, have particular diets, etc.

Admonish bad self talk. If your daughter starts in on themselves, or states she looks bad in something, put a stop to it right away. If you let her carry on you're giving her permission to have a bad body image. You're almost telling her you agree with her assessment, and you're letting a bad cycle perpetuate.

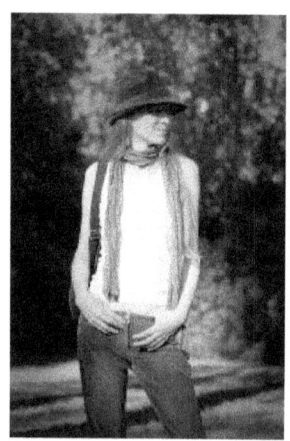

Wrapping Up

Body image is something that we likely have all fought with at one time or other. Even those gifted with exceptional genetics have insecurities about their bodies. These insecurities, when brooded on, tend to fester, and may lead to really serious issues. Damaging body image isn't something to be taken lightly. If your daughter has a bad body image now, it may impact things you'll do years from now. It's crucial to realize the risks of bad body images, and help your girls to defeat this inclination, and be positive about who they are and how they appear.

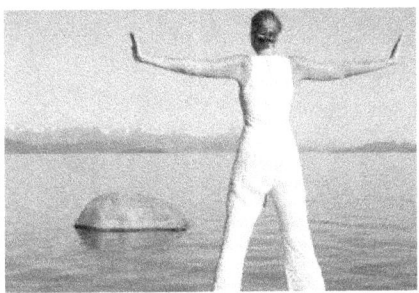

www.ingramcontent.com/pod-product-compliance
Lightning Source LLC
Chambersburg PA
CBHW070801180526
45168CB00004B/1704